CONTENTS

CHAPTER ONE — 1
CHAPTER TWO — 5
CHAPTER THREE — 9
CHAPTER FOUR — 18
CHAPTER FIVE — 22
CHAPTER SIX — 27
CHAPTER SEVEN — 32
CHAPTER EIGHT — 35
CHAPTER EIGHT — 40
CHAPTER NINE — 62

CHAPTER ONE

INTRODUCTION

EXPLORING THE BLUE ZONE DIET

The Blue Zone diet is a fascinating concept that has been gaining popularity in recent years due to its association with longevity and improved overall health. In this article, we will delve into the essence of the Blue Zone diet, why it has been gaining traction, the numerous health benefits it offers, and its ultimate purpose and goals.

Brief Explanation of the Blue Zone Diet Concept

The Blue Zone diet takes its name from the term "Blue Zones," which refers to regions around the world where people tend to live significantly longer and healthier lives compared to the global average. These regions include places like Okinawa in Japan, Sardinia in Italy, Nicoya in Costa Rica, Ikaria in Greece, and Loma Linda in California.

The core idea behind the Blue Zone diet is to adopt the dietary patterns and lifestyle habits of these long-lived populations. These diets are primarily plant-based, with a strong emphasis on locally sourced, whole, and unprocessed foods. They typically consist of vegetables, fruits, legumes, whole grains, and nuts. Fish and lean meats are consumed in moderation, while processed foods, sugar, and excessive amounts of dairy and red meat are avoided.

One of the key principles of the Blue Zone diet is mindful eating. It encourages people to savor their meals, eat slowly, and stop when they are 80% full. This practice not only helps with portion control but also promotes a deeper connection with food and satisfaction after eating.

Why the Blue Zone Diet Is Gaining Popularity

The Blue Zone diet has been gaining popularity for several compelling reasons:

1. **Longevity and Health:** People are increasingly drawn to the promise of a longer and healthier life. With the rising interest in wellness and anti-aging strategies, the Blue Zone diet offers a practical approach backed by real-world examples of success.

2. **Scientific Support:** Research has provided substantial evidence supporting the health benefits of the Blue Zone diet. Studies have shown that these diets can reduce the risk of chronic diseases such as heart disease, diabetes, and cancer, which are major concerns in many parts of the world.

3. **Cultural Appeal:** The Blue Zone diet draws from the culinary traditions of diverse cultures, making it accessible and appealing to a wide range of people. It celebrates the joy of communal meals and the use of fresh, seasonal ingredients.

4. **Sustainability:** The emphasis on plant-based foods and local sourcing aligns with the growing awareness of the environmental impact of food production. Many individuals are choosing this diet as a way to reduce their carbon footprint.

The Health Benefits Associated with the Blue Zone Diet

The health benefits of the Blue Zone diet are numerous and extend beyond just longevity:

1. **Heart Health:** The diet's focus on plant-based foods, high fiber content, and healthy fats can lower the risk of heart disease. It also promotes healthy cholesterol levels and blood pressure.

2. **Weight Management:** The Blue Zone diet's mindful eating approach helps with weight control. By eating slowly and stopping when satisfied, individuals are less likely to overeat.

3. **Improved Digestion:** The diet's rich fiber content from fruits, vegetables, and whole grains promotes healthy digestion and regular bowel movements.

4. **Mental Well-being:** Nutrient-dense foods in the Blue Zone diet provide essential vitamins and minerals that support brain health. Additionally, the social aspect of communal meals contributes to reduced stress and increased happiness.

5. **Reduced Inflammation:** The anti-inflammatory properties of many Blue Zone diet components can help mitigate chronic inflammation, a key factor in various diseases.

The Purpose and Goal of the Blue Zone Diet

The ultimate purpose of the Blue Zone diet is to enable individuals to lead longer, healthier, and more fulfilling lives. Its primary goals can be summarized as follows:

- **Increase Longevity:** By adopting the dietary and lifestyle practices of Blue Zone regions, individuals aim to extend their lifespan and maintain good health well into old age.

- **Enhance Quality of Life:** The diet seeks to improve the overall quality of life by reducing the risk of chronic diseases and promoting physical and mental well-being.

- **Cultural Preservation:** The Blue Zone diet celebrates cultural diversity and traditions related to food. It encourages the preservation of culinary heritage and the enjoyment of locally sourced, seasonal ingredients.

- **Environmental Sustainability:** By prioritizing plant-based foods and local sourcing, the Blue Zone diet aligns with the goal of minimizing the environmental impact of food production.

In conclusion, the Blue Zone diet represents a holistic approach to well-being, drawing inspiration from some of the world's healthiest and longest-lived populations.

CHAPTER TWO

UNDERSTANDING THE BLUE ZONE DIET

Exploring the Origins and Principles of the Blue Zone Diet:

The Blue Zone diet is a dietary pattern associated with regions of the world where people have notably long and healthy lives. These regions are known as Blue Zones, and they include places like Okinawa (Japan), Sardinia (Italy), Nicoya (Costa Rica), Ikaria (Greece), and Loma Linda (California, USA). The term "Blue Zone" was coined by Dan Buettner, a National Geographic fellow who identified and studied these regions.

The Blue Zone diet is based on the observation that people in these regions tend to share certain dietary and lifestyle habits that contribute to their longevity. Some of the key principles of the Blue Zone diet include:

1. **Plant-Based Foods:** Blue Zone diets are predominantly plant-based. People in these regions consume a variety of fruits, vegetables, legumes, nuts, and whole grains. These foods are rich in essential nutrients, fiber, and antioxidants, which can promote good health and longevity.

2. **Moderation:** Blue Zone populations practice

portion control and moderation when it comes to their meals. They eat until they are satisfied but not overly full, which can help prevent overeating and obesity.

3. **Limited Meat Consumption:** While not strictly vegetarian, the Blue Zone diet places a strong emphasis on limiting meat consumption, especially red meat. Instead, they opt for lean sources of protein such as fish and occasionally small amounts of poultry. This dietary choice is believed to reduce the risk of chronic diseases associated with excessive meat consumption.

4. **Beans and Legumes:** Legumes like beans, lentils, and chickpeas are staples in Blue Zone diets. They are excellent sources of protein, fiber, and various vitamins and minerals. Consuming legumes regularly can have numerous health benefits.

The Science Behind the Blue Zone Diet and Its Impact on Longevity:

The Blue Zone diet's impact on longevity is backed by scientific research and has several explanations:

1. Nutrient Density: The plant-based foods found in Blue Zone diets are rich in essential nutrients and antioxidants, which can reduce inflammation and oxidative stress, potentially slowing down the aging process and lowering the risk of chronic diseases.

2. Fiber Content: High-fiber diets from whole grains and vegetables promote digestive health, regulate blood sugar levels, and help maintain a healthy weight, all of which are factors associated with

longevity.

3. Healthy Fats: Blue Zone diets often include sources of healthy fats, such as olive oil and nuts, which can support heart health and overall well-being.

4. Social and Lifestyle Factors: Blue Zone communities prioritize strong social connections, physical activity, and a sense of purpose, which contribute to reduced stress and better mental health, further enhancing longevity.

Debunking Common Misconceptions About the Blue Zone Diet:

1. **It's a Strict Vegetarian Diet:** While Blue Zone diets are primarily plant-based, they are not necessarily vegetarian. Some Blue Zone populations do include small amounts of animal products, but these are typically consumed in moderation.

2. **It's a One-Size-Fits-All Diet:** The Blue Zone diet is not a rigid diet plan but a set of principles. It can be adapted to individual preferences and cultural variations while still promoting health and longevity.

3. **It Guarantees Longevity:** The Blue Zone diet is just one factor contributing to the long and healthy lives of these populations. Lifestyle factors, genetics, and the environment also play significant roles.

In conclusion, the Blue Zone diet emphasizes plant-based foods, moderation, and limited meat consumption as key components. Scientific evidence suggests that these dietary principles, combined with a holistic lifestyle approach, can contribute to longevity and better health.

CHAPTER THREE

BLUE ZONE DIET STAPLES

A Detailed List of Foods Commonly Found in Blue Zone Regions

Blue Zones are regions of the world where people tend to live longer and healthier lives. The longevity and well-being of these communities have been attributed to their unique diets, among other factors. In this section, we will explore the foods commonly found in Blue Zone regions and how they contribute to the health and vitality of their residents.

1. Leafy Greens

Leafy greens are a staple in Blue Zone diets. Varieties like kale, spinach, and collard greens are packed with essential nutrients, including vitamins A, C, and K, as well as folate and fiber. These greens are not only nutrient-dense but also low in calories, making them a key component of a balanced diet.

2. Beans and Legumes

Beans and legumes, such as lentils, chickpeas, and black beans, are rich in plant-based protein, fiber, and complex carbohydrates. They provide sustained energy, help regulate blood sugar levels, and contribute to a feeling of fullness, reducing the risk of overeating.

3. Whole Grains

Blue Zone inhabitants consume whole grains like quinoa, barley, and brown rice, which are excellent sources of fiber, vitamins, and minerals. Whole grains promote heart health, aid in digestion, and maintain stable energy levels throughout the day.

4. Nuts and Seeds

Almonds, walnuts, and flaxseeds are among the nuts and seeds prevalent in Blue Zone diets. They offer healthy fats, protein, and a variety of vitamins and minerals. These snacks not only satisfy hunger but also support brain health and reduce the risk of chronic diseases.

5. Fruits

Blue Zone regions are abundant in fruits like blueberries, apples, and oranges. These fruits are loaded with antioxidants, vitamins, and dietary fiber, which are essential for overall health and disease prevention.

6. Fish

In coastal Blue Zone areas, fish is a dietary mainstay. Fish, particularly fatty varieties like salmon and mackerel, provide omega-3 fatty acids, which are known to promote heart health and reduce inflammation.

7. Olive Oil

Olive oil is a cornerstone of Blue Zone cuisine. It is rich in monounsaturated fats, which support cardiovascular health, and contains antioxidants that combat oxidative stress. Olive oil is often used as a healthy cooking oil and salad dressing.

8. Herbs and Spices

Herbs and spices add flavor and depth to Blue Zone dishes without the need for excessive salt or unhealthy fats. Commonly used herbs include rosemary, oregano, and basil, while spices like turmeric and cinnamon offer various health benefits.

9. Water

Proper hydration is crucial for health, and Blue Zone residents typically drink plenty of water throughout the day. Staying well-hydrated supports digestion, circulation, and overall vitality.

10. Red Wine (in moderation)

Some Blue Zone communities enjoy red wine in moderation. Red wine contains resveratrol, an antioxidant that may contribute to heart health. However, it's essential to consume alcohol in moderation to reap the potential benefits without the risks.

Incorporating these foods into your diet, as inspired by Blue Zone regions, can promote longevity and well-being. Their nutrient-rich, plant-based nature aligns with principles of balanced nutrition, making them a valuable addition to anyone's dietary habits.

How to Incorporate Legumes, Whole Grains, and Nuts into Your Daily Diet

Legumes, whole grains, and nuts are nutrient powerhouses that can enhance your diet's nutritional profile and contribute to your overall health. Here, we'll explore various ways to incorporate these wholesome foods into your daily meals.

Legumes

1. **Bean Salads**: Create colorful salads by mixing

different types of beans, such as kidney beans, black beans, and chickpeas, with fresh vegetables, herbs, and a light vinaigrette.

2. **Hummus**: Make homemade hummus by blending chickpeas, tahini, lemon juice, and garlic. Enjoy it as a dip with whole-grain pita bread or as a spread in sandwiches.

3. **Lentil Soups**: Prepare hearty lentil soups with a mix of vegetables and spices for a warm and satisfying meal.

4. **Bean Burritos**: Fill whole-grain tortillas with black beans, brown rice, and your favorite toppings for a nutritious and flavorful burrito.

5. **Bean-based Pasta**: Explore pasta made from legume flours like lentil or chickpea pasta, which offer added protein and fiber.

Whole Grains

1. **Oatmeal**: Start your day with a bowl of oatmeal topped with fresh fruits, nuts, and a drizzle of honey for a wholesome breakfast.

2. **Quinoa Salad**: Create a refreshing quinoa salad with diced vegetables, herbs, and a light lemon dressing for a nutritious side dish.

3. **Brown Rice Bowls**: Build customizable rice bowls with brown rice as the base and a variety of vegetables, lean protein, and flavorful sauces.

4. **Whole Wheat Bread**: Choose whole wheat or whole grain bread for sandwiches and toast to increase your whole grain intake.

5. **Barley Risotto**: Experiment with barley as a

substitute for Arborio rice in a creamy, vegetable-packed risotto.

Nuts

1. **Trail Mix**: Prepare a homemade trail mix by combining almonds, walnuts, dried fruits, and dark chocolate chips for a satisfying snack.

2. **Nut Butter**: Spread almond or peanut butter on whole grain toast or use it as a dip for apple slices or celery sticks.

3. **Nut-Encrusted Protein**: Coat chicken or fish with crushed nuts and bake for a crunchy, protein-rich main course.

4. **Yogurt Parfait**: Layer Greek yogurt with mixed berries and a sprinkle of chopped nuts for a nutrient-packed dessert.

5. **Smoothie Boost**: Add a spoonful of nut butter or a handful of nuts to your morning smoothie for extra creaminess and nutrition.

Incorporating legumes, whole grains, and nuts into your daily diet can improve your overall well-being by providing essential nutrients, fiber, and healthy fats. These versatile foods offer a wide range of options for creating delicious and nutritious meals, making it easier to prioritize your health.

The Importance of Olive Oil and Its Health Benefits

Olive oil, often referred to as "liquid gold," has been a fundamental component of the Mediterranean diet for centuries. Its importance in promoting health and well-being cannot be overstated. Here, we'll explore the significance of olive oil and its numerous health benefits.

Heart Health

One of the primary reasons olive oil is celebrated is its heart-protective properties. It is rich in monounsaturated fats, specifically oleic acid, which has been linked to improved cardiovascular health. Consuming olive oil regularly can help reduce the risk of heart disease by lowering bad cholesterol levels and promoting healthy blood vessel function.

Anti-Inflammatory Properties

Olive oil contains potent antioxidants, such as vitamin E and polyphenols, that combat oxidative stress and inflammation in the body. This anti-inflammatory effect may contribute to a reduced risk of chronic diseases, including cancer and arthritis.

Weight Management

Contrary to the misconception that all fats lead to weight gain, olive oil can support weight management when used in moderation. Its healthy fats help increase feelings of fullness, reducing the likelihood of overeating.

Digestive Health

Olive oil can aid in digestion by promoting the production of bile, which aids in the breakdown of fats. It also has a mild laxative effect, which can help prevent constipation.

Brain Health

The monounsaturated fats in olive oil have been associated with improved cognitive function and a reduced risk of age-related cognitive decline. Including olive oil in your diet may support brain health and memory.

Skin and Hair Health

Olive oil's moisturizing and antioxidant properties make it beneficial for skin and hair. It can be applied topically as a natural moisturizer or used in homemade beauty treatments.

Versatility in Cooking

Olive oil's versatility extends to the kitchen. It can be used for sautéing, roasting, grilling, and as a dressing for salads. Its rich flavor enhances the taste of a wide variety of dishes.

Quality Matters

To reap the full benefits of olive oil, it's essential to choose high-quality, extra-virgin olive oil. Look for certifications and opt for oils that come in dark glass bottles to protect against light exposure.

Incorporating olive oil into your diet can be a flavorful and health-conscious choice. Whether drizzled over a salad, used for cooking, or simply enjoyed with a slice of whole-grain bread, olive oil is a valuable addition to any culinary repertoire.

The Role of Herbs and Spices in Blue Zone Cuisine

Herbs and spices play a significant role in Blue Zone cuisine, adding depth, flavor, and health benefits to dishes. Let's delve into the importance of herbs and spices in these longevity-promoting diets.

Flavor Enhancement

Herbs and spices are natural flavor enhancers that can elevate the taste of even the simplest dishes. They provide complexity and depth without the need for excessive salt, sugar, or unhealthy fats.

Nutritional Value

Many herbs and spices are packed with essential nutrients, including vitamins, minerals, and antioxidants. For example, cinnamon is rich in antioxidants, while fresh herbs like parsley and cilantro provide vitamins A and C.

Digestive Health

Certain herbs and spices, such as ginger and mint, have digestive benefits. They can alleviate indigestion, bloating, and nausea when incorporated into meals or consumed as herbal teas.

Anti-Inflammatory Properties

Turmeric, a vibrant spice often used in Blue Zone cuisine, contains curcumin, a potent anti-inflammatory compound. Regular consumption of turmeric may help reduce the risk of chronic diseases associated with inflammation.

Antioxidant Power

Herbs and spices are among the most antioxidant-rich foods available. They help combat oxidative stress and protect the body's cells from damage caused by free radicals.

Cultural Significance

Herbs and spices are integral to the cultural heritage of Blue Zone regions. They have been used for generations in traditional recipes, preserving culinary traditions that contribute to community well-being.

Balanced Seasoning

Using herbs and spices allows for more balanced seasoning in dishes. This promotes healthier eating habits by reducing the reliance on excessive salt or sugar.

Variety and Creativity

The vast array of herbs and spices available encourages culinary experimentation and creativity. It enables cooks to develop unique and delicious dishes while reaping the health benefits of these natural ingredients.

CHAPTER FOUR

KEY FOODS IN THE BLUE ZONE DIET

The Blue Zone Diet is renowned for its ability to promote longevity and overall well-being. This dietary pattern has gained significant attention due to its association with communities where people tend to live longer, healthier lives. The key foods in the Blue Zone Diet contribute significantly to this exceptional longevity. Let's delve into the primary components of this dietary regimen.

Beans and Legumes

Beans and legumes are the cornerstone of the Blue Zone Diet. These nutrient-dense foods are packed with fiber, protein, and essential vitamins and minerals. Varieties like chickpeas, lentils, and black beans are frequently consumed in Blue Zone regions. They provide a steady source of energy, help maintain a healthy weight, and support digestive health.

Points to Note:

1. **Rich in Protein:** Beans and legumes are an excellent plant-based source of protein, making them a staple for vegetarians and vegans.

2. **Fiber-Rich:** The high fiber content helps regulate blood sugar levels and lowers the risk of heart disease.

3. **Antioxidant Powerhouse:** They contain antioxidants that combat inflammation and oxidative stress.

Whole Grains

Whole grains are another fundamental component of the Blue Zone Diet. These include foods like brown rice, quinoa, oats, and whole wheat. Whole grains are rich in fiber, vitamins, and minerals, making them essential for maintaining good health.

Points to Note:

1. **Fiber Boost:** Whole grains provide a significant fiber boost, aiding in digestion and promoting a feeling of fullness.

2. **Heart Health:** They help reduce the risk of heart disease by lowering cholesterol levels and maintaining healthy blood pressure.

3. **Nutrient-Rich:** Whole grains are packed with nutrients like B vitamins, iron, and magnesium.

Fruits and Vegetables

A colorful array of fruits and vegetables is a hallmark of the Blue Zone Diet. These foods are not only visually appealing but also incredibly nutritious. Berries, leafy greens, tomatoes, and sweet potatoes are commonly consumed in Blue Zones.

Points to Note:

1. **Abundant Vitamins and Minerals:** Fruits and vegetables provide essential vitamins and minerals that support overall health.

2. **Antioxidant-Rich:** They are brimming with

antioxidants, protecting cells from damage and reducing the risk of chronic diseases.

3. **Hydration:** Fruits and vegetables are high in water content, aiding in hydration and promoting radiant skin.

Nuts and Seeds

Nuts and seeds are small powerhouses of nutrition in the Blue Zone Diet. Almonds, walnuts, chia seeds, and flaxseeds are often incorporated into meals and snacks. They are a source of healthy fats, protein, and various vitamins and minerals.

Points to Note:

1. **Healthy Fats:** Nuts and seeds provide essential fatty acids that support brain health and reduce the risk of heart disease.

2. **Satiety:** The combination of healthy fats and protein helps keep you feeling full and satisfied.

3. **Bone Health:** Some nuts and seeds, like almonds, are rich in calcium, promoting strong bones.

Herbs and Spices

Herbs and spices are used generously in Blue Zone cuisine to enhance flavor without relying on excessive salt or sugar. Common herbs include rosemary, basil, and oregano, while spices like turmeric and cinnamon are also valued for their health benefits.

Points to Note:

1. **Reduced Sodium Intake:** Herbs and spices allow for flavorful dishes with less sodium, which is beneficial for heart health.

2. **Anti-Inflammatory:** Many herbs and spices possess anti-inflammatory properties, reducing the risk of chronic diseases.

3. **Metabolism Boost:** Some spices, like cinnamon, may help improve insulin sensitivity and metabolism.

Fermented Food

Fermented foods, such as yogurt, kefir, sauerkraut, and kimchi, are consumed in Blue Zones for their probiotic content. These foods promote a healthy gut microbiome, which plays a crucial role in overall well-being.

Points to Note:

1. **Digestive Health:** Fermented foods support a balanced gut microbiome, aiding digestion and nutrient absorption.

2. **Immune Support:** Probiotics in fermented foods strengthen the immune system, reducing the risk of infections.

3. **Mood and Mental Health:** There is emerging evidence that a healthy gut can positively impact mood and mental health.

CHAPTER FIVE

MEAL PLANNING AND PREPARATION
Tips for Effective Meal Planning on the Blue Zone Diet

Meal planning on the Blue Zone diet is a powerful tool for promoting longevity and overall well-being. To make the most of this dietary approach, consider the following tips:

1. **Embrace Plant-Based Foods**: The foundation of the Blue Zone diet is plant-based foods like vegetables, fruits, legumes, and whole grains. Aim to fill the majority of your plate with these nutritious options.

2. **Incorporate Beans and Lentils**: Beans and lentils are rich sources of protein and fiber. They are staples in Blue Zone regions and should be a regular part of your meals.

3. **Limit Meat Consumption**: Red meat is consumed sparingly in Blue Zone diets. Opt for leaner protein sources like fish, poultry, or tofu instead.

4. **Choose Healthy Fats**: Use olive oil as your primary cooking oil, and include nuts and seeds in your diet for healthy fats. These fats are associated with reduced risk of heart disease.

5. **Eat a Rainbow of Fruits and Vegetables**: Different colors of fruits and vegetables provide various

nutrients. Try to include a variety of colors in your meals to ensure a wide range of vitamins and minerals.

6. **Whole Grains Are Key**: Opt for whole grains like brown rice, quinoa, and whole wheat pasta over refined grains. They offer more fiber and nutrients.

7. **Moderate Dairy Consumption**: If you consume dairy, choose low-fat options like Greek yogurt and cheese in moderation. Blue Zone communities often consume dairy in smaller quantities.

8. **Stay Hydrated**: Water is essential for overall health. Drink plenty of water throughout the day, and consider herbal teas or infused water for added flavor.

9. **Mindful Eating**: Pay attention to portion sizes and eat slowly. This helps prevent overeating and promotes better digestion.

10. **Plan Ahead**: Plan your meals for the week ahead of time. This will help you make healthier choices and reduce the temptation to opt for fast food or unhealthy snacks.

Sample Blue Zone Diet Meal Plans

Breakfast

- **Oatmeal**: Top a bowl of steel-cut oats with fresh berries, chopped nuts, and a drizzle of honey.

- **Smoothie**: Blend spinach, banana, almond milk, and a spoonful of almond butter for a nutritious morning shake.

- **Fruit Salad**: Combine a variety of seasonal fruits like oranges, apples, and kiwi for a refreshing breakfast.

Lunch

- **Mediterranean Salad**: Create a salad with mixed greens, cherry tomatoes, cucumber, olives, and feta cheese. Dress it with olive oil and balsamic vinegar.

- **Quinoa Bowl**: Cook quinoa and top it with grilled vegetables, chickpeas, and a tahini dressing.

- **Vegetable Stir-Fry**: Sauté a mix of colorful vegetables in olive oil and garlic, then serve over brown rice.

Dinner

- **Grilled Fish**: Grill a piece of salmon or cod and serve it with a side of steamed broccoli and quinoa.

- **Lentil Stew**: Make a hearty stew with lentils, carrots, celery, and tomatoes. Season with herbs and spices for flavor.

- **Tofu and Vegetable Skewers**: Marinate tofu and a variety of vegetables in a flavorful sauce, then grill until tender.

Cooking Techniques and Recipes for the Blue Zone Diet

To align your cooking with Blue Zone principles, consider the following techniques and recipes:

Cooking Techniques

- **Steaming**: Steaming vegetables helps retain their

nutrients. Use a steamer basket or a microwave-safe dish with a lid.

- **Baking and Roasting**: Bake or roast vegetables and lean proteins like chicken or fish with minimal added fats for a delicious, healthy meal.

- **Stir-Frying**: Quickly cook vegetables in a hot pan with a small amount of olive oil and a dash of soy sauce for a tasty stir-fry.

- **Poaching**: Poach eggs or poultry in simmering water with herbs and spices for a flavorful, low-fat dish.

Blue Zone Recipes

- **Minestrone Soup**: A hearty soup made with vegetables, beans, and whole wheat pasta. Season with basil and oregano.

- **Greek Salad**: Combine cucumbers, tomatoes, red onions, olives, and feta cheese. Dress with olive oil and lemon juice.

- **Ratatouille**: A classic Provençal dish with eggplant, tomatoes, bell peppers, zucchini, and aromatic herbs.

Creating Balanced and Satisfying Blue Zone Meals

Balanced and satisfying Blue Zone meals should include the following elements:

1. **Plant-Based Foods**: Make vegetables, fruits, and whole grains the centerpiece of your meal.

2. **Protein**: Incorporate lean protein sources such as beans, lentils, tofu, fish, or poultry.

3. **Healthy Fats**: Include sources of healthy fats like olive oil, nuts, and seeds.

4. **Fiber**: Ensure your meal is rich in fiber from whole grains and vegetables to promote digestion and fullness.

5. **Variety**: Aim for a variety of colors, flavors, and textures on your plate to make the meal enjoyable.

6. **Portion Control**: Pay attention to portion sizes to avoid overeating.

7. **Hydration**: Complement your meal with water, herbal tea, or infused water.

8. **Mindful Eating**: Eat slowly and savor each bite to appreciate the flavors and prevent overconsumption.

CHAPTER SIX

BLUE ZONE DIET RECIPES

Exploring the Blue Zone Lifestyle through Delicious Recipes

The Blue Zones have long fascinated researchers and health enthusiasts alike. These unique regions around the world are known for their populations' exceptional longevity and good health. One of the key factors contributing to this longevity is their diet. In this section, we'll delve into a collection of delicious and nutritious Blue Zone recipes that offer a glimpse into the secrets of a longer, healthier life.

A Collection of Delicious and Nutritious Blue Zone Recipes

The Blue Zone regions, which include areas in Greece, Italy, Japan, and Costa Rica, share common dietary patterns. Their diets are primarily plant-based, emphasizing vegetables, legumes, whole grains, and nuts. These ingredients form the foundation of various mouthwatering dishes.

Mediterranean Delights

1. **Mediterranean Vegetable Stew:** Start with a base of tomatoes, peppers, and eggplants, then add chickpeas, onions, and a medley of herbs. Slow-cook until the flavors meld together, resulting in a hearty stew.

2. **Greek Salad:** This classic salad combines fresh cucumbers, tomatoes, olives, and feta cheese, drizzled with olive oil and sprinkled with oregano. It's a refreshing and nutrient-packed dish.

3. **Hummus and Tzatziki:** These creamy dips, made from chickpeas and yogurt, are perfect for dipping fresh vegetables or whole-grain pita bread.

Japanese Elegance

1. **Miso Soup:** A comforting and savory soup made from fermented soybean paste, seaweed, and tofu. It's both flavorful and packed with probiotics.

2. **Sushi Rolls:** Create your own sushi rolls with brown rice, fresh vegetables, and a touch of wasabi. It's a fun and healthy way to enjoy the flavors of Japan.

Costa Rican Simplicity

1. **Gallo Pinto:** This traditional Costa Rican dish features black beans and rice, often served with a side of plantains. It's a simple yet satisfying meal.

2. **Casado:** A typical Costa Rican plate that includes rice, beans, vegetables, and a choice of protein like grilled chicken or fish. It's a balanced and nutritious option.

Breakfast Options that Promote Longevity

Breakfast is often considered the most important meal of the day, and the Blue Zone inhabitants have their own unique morning rituals that contribute to their long lives.

Oatmeal with a Twist

1. **Muesli:** A blend of rolled oats, nuts, dried fruits, and yogurt, muesli provides a hearty and

nutrient-rich start to the day.

2. **Greek Yogurt Parfait:** Layer Greek yogurt with honey, berries, and granola for a protein-packed and delicious breakfast.

Japanese Elegance

1. **Tamago Sando:** A Japanese egg sandwich made with fluffy omelets and a touch of mayo. It's a delightful fusion of flavors.

2. **Natto and Rice:** Natto, fermented soybeans, is a staple in Japan and is often enjoyed with steamed rice and a drizzle of soy sauce.

Blue Zone-Inspired Salads, Soups, and Stews

Salads, soups, and stews are essential components of Blue Zone diets, offering a plethora of nutrients and flavors.

The Mediterranean Way

1. **Greek Lentil Soup:** A hearty soup made from lentils, tomatoes, and vegetables. It's a comforting dish packed with fiber and protein.

2. **Tabbouleh Salad:** A refreshing salad featuring bulgur, parsley, mint, tomatoes, and cucumbers, dressed with lemon juice and olive oil.

Japanese Comfort

1. **Miso Udon Soup:** A warming bowl of udon noodles in miso broth, garnished with scallions and seaweed.

2. **Edamame Salad:** Steamed edamame beans, tossed with sesame oil, sesame seeds, and a dash of soy sauce. It's a simple yet satisfying salad.

Entrees Featuring Plant-Based Proteins and Lean Meats

The Blue Zone diet is characterized by a limited consumption of meat, with a focus on plant-based proteins and lean cuts when meat is included.

Plant-Powered Plates

1. **Tofu Stir-Fry:** Cubes of tofu sautéed with an assortment of vegetables and a flavorful stir-fry sauce. It's a protein-packed and colorful dish.

2. **Chickpea Curry:** A fragrant and spicy curry made with chickpeas, tomatoes, and a blend of aromatic spices. It's a vegetarian delight.

Lean Meats in Moderation

1. **Grilled Fish:** Blue Zone regions near the sea often feature grilled fish like sardines or mackerel, rich in omega-3 fatty acids and protein.

2. **Chicken Souvlaki:** Marinated and grilled chicken skewers served with a side of pita bread and fresh vegetables. It's a balanced and delicious meal.

Desserts and Snacks that are Blue Zone-Friendly

Even in the Blue Zones, there's room for indulgence, albeit in moderation. Here are some sweet treats and snacks that align with the principles of Blue Zone living.

Sweet Temptations

1. **Fresh Fruit Salad:** A medley of ripe, seasonal fruits drizzled with honey or a sprinkle of cinnamon. It's a guilt-free dessert.

2. **Yogurt with Honey:** Creamy Greek yogurt topped with a drizzle of honey and a handful of crushed nuts. It's a simple yet satisfying dessert.

Healthy Snack Choices

1. **Mixed Nuts:** A handful of mixed nuts, such as almonds, walnuts, and pistachios, provide healthy fats and a satisfying crunch.

2. **Baked Sweet Potato Fries:** Sliced sweet potatoes tossed in olive oil and baked until crispy. They're a nutritious alternative to traditional fries.

CHAPTER SEVEN

INCORPORATING BLUE ZONE DIET INTO YOUR LIFESTYLE

Transitioning to a Blue Zone diet, which is based on the eating habits of people in regions known for longevity and good health, can be a positive step towards improving your overall well-being. Here are some strategies to help you make the transition, shop for ingredients, dine out, and stay motivated:

1. **Gradual Diet Changes:**
   - Start gradually by incorporating one or two Blue Zone principles at a time.
   - Focus on increasing your intake of plant-based foods like fruits, vegetables, whole grains, and legumes.
   - Reduce your consumption of processed foods, sugary drinks, and unhealthy fats.

2. **How to Shop for Blue Zone Ingredients:**
   - Prioritize fresh, seasonal, and locally sourced produce.
   - Look for whole grains like quinoa, brown rice, and whole wheat pasta.
   - Buy a variety of beans, lentils, and chickpeas for protein.

- Choose nuts and seeds such as almonds, walnuts, and chia seeds.
- Opt for herbs and spices like basil, oregano, and turmeric to flavor dishes.

3. **Making Informed Choices:**
    - Read food labels to avoid products with high levels of added sugars, trans fats, and artificial ingredients.
    - Choose olive oil as your primary cooking fat and for salad dressings.
    - Prioritize organic and pesticide-free options when possible.
    - Consider buying in bulk to reduce packaging waste.

4. **Dining Out on the Blue Zone Diet:**
    - Look for restaurants that offer plant-based options or Mediterranean-style dishes.
    - Request dishes with extra vegetables and legumes.
    - Avoid fried and heavily processed menu items.
    - Ask for sauces and dressings on the side to control portions.

5. **Staying Motivated and Maintaining a Healthy Blue Zone Lifestyle:**
    - Find a community or support group that shares your dietary goals.
    - Experiment with Blue Zone recipes and cooking techniques to keep meals

exciting.

- Plan your meals and snacks in advance to prevent unhealthy food choices when you're hungry.

- Reflect on the health benefits and longevity associated with the Blue Zone diet to stay motivated.

CHAPTER EIGHT

SUCCESS STORIES

Exploring Real-life Stories of Blue Zone Diet Enthusiasts

The Blue Zone diet has gained significant attention in recent years for its potential to promote longevity and overall well-being. In this section, we will delve into the real-life stories of individuals who have wholeheartedly embraced the Blue Zone diet, sharing their experiences, health improvements, and the valuable lessons they have learned along the way.

A Journey to Vibrant Health

Meet Sarah, a 52-year-old accountant from Loma Linda, California, one of the famous Blue Zones. She decided to adopt the Blue Zone diet after witnessing her parents' struggle with age-related health issues. Sarah was determined to take a proactive approach to her health and longevity. She began incorporating the principles of the Blue Zone diet into her daily life, focusing on plant-based foods, whole grains, and minimal meat consumption.

Over the course of a year, Sarah noticed remarkable changes in her health. Her energy levels surged, and she shed excess weight without counting calories or following fad diets. Sarah's cholesterol levels dropped, and her blood pressure stabilized. Most notably, she felt a profound sense of vitality that she hadn't experienced in years.

Key Takeaways:

- Sarah's journey illustrates the power of the Blue Zone diet in promoting overall health and vitality.

- Her experience highlights the significance of making gradual dietary changes for long-lasting results.

Overcoming Health Challenges

John, a 64-year-old retired teacher from Ikaria, Greece, had struggled with high blood pressure and joint pain for years. Frustrated with the side effects of medications, he decided to explore alternative approaches to improve his health. After learning about the Blue Zone diet, he decided to give it a try.

John gradually transitioned to a diet rich in fruits, vegetables, and whole grains while reducing his consumption of processed foods. Within a few months, he began to experience remarkable improvements. His blood pressure normalized, and his joint pain significantly decreased. He also found that he was sleeping better and waking up with a newfound sense of vitality.

Key Takeaways:

- John's story demonstrates how the Blue Zone diet can offer effective solutions for managing chronic health conditions.

- It underscores the importance of personalized dietary choices for optimal results.

The Blue Zone Diet: Lessons Learned and Health Improvements

In this section, we will further explore the lessons learned by individuals who have embraced the Blue Zone diet, as well as the notable health improvements they have experienced.

The Power of Community

One common thread among Blue Zone communities is the emphasis on social connections and a sense of belonging. Martha, a 58-year-old resident of Sardinia, Italy, noted that the act of sharing meals with friends and family became a central part of her life after adopting the Blue Zone diet. She found that this sense of community contributed significantly to her overall well-being.

Martha's experience highlights the importance of not only what we eat but also how we eat it. The Blue Zone diet encourages communal dining and fosters strong bonds, which can positively impact mental and emotional health.

Key Takeaways:

- Martha's story underscores the significance of communal dining and social connections in the Blue Zone lifestyle.

- It reminds us that the way we consume our meals can be as crucial as the foods themselves.

Sustainable Health and Longevity

David, a 70-year-old retired engineer from Nicoya, Costa Rica, is a testament to the sustainable nature of the Blue Zone diet. He has been following this lifestyle for over a decade and continues to enjoy excellent health. David's story serves as a reminder that the Blue Zone diet is not a quick fix but a long-term commitment to well-being.

Through his journey, David has learned that the key to success is consistency. He emphasizes the importance of making the Blue Zone diet a part of your daily routine, not just a temporary diet. This approach has allowed him to maintain his vitality and quality of life well into his senior years.

Key Takeaways:

- David's experience highlights the longevity of the Blue Zone diet when integrated into one's daily life.

- It encourages individuals to view the diet as a sustainable lifestyle choice.

Inspirational Anecdotes Showcasing the Benefits of the Blue Zone Diet

The Blue Zone diet offers not only physical health benefits but also a profound sense of well-being. In this section, we'll explore inspirational anecdotes that showcase the transformative power of this dietary lifestyle.

Rediscovering the Joy of Life

Elena, a 48-year-old artist from Okinawa, Japan, found herself in a creative rut for years. She was overweight and lacked the energy and inspiration to pursue her artistic passions. After embracing the Blue Zone diet, she experienced a remarkable transformation.

As Elena's health improved, she discovered a newfound zest for life. Her weight stabilized, and her energy levels soared. With renewed vitality, she began creating art like never before, drawing inspiration from the vibrant, plant-based foods that had become a staple of her diet.

Key Takeaways:

- Elena's story illustrates how the Blue Zone diet

can rekindle passion and creativity in life.

- It reminds us that vibrant health extends beyond physical well-being to encompass emotional and creative fulfillment.

Thriving in Later Years

Richard, an 82-year-old resident of Nicoya, Costa Rica, is a testament to the idea that age is just a number. He credits his longevity and vitality to the Blue Zone diet he has followed for decades. Richard continues to engage in physical activities, tend to his garden, and enjoy the company of his grandchildren.

Richard's story serves as an inspiration to all who seek to age gracefully. It showcases the remarkable potential of the Blue Zone diet to not only extend life but also enhance its quality in later years.

Key Takeaways:

- Richard's experience demonstrates that age doesn't have to limit one's quality of life.

- It highlights the profound impact of the Blue Zone diet on overall well-being, even in the later stages of life.

In conclusion, the real-life stories of individuals who have embraced the Blue Zone diet provide compelling evidence of its transformative power

CHAPTER EIGHT

RECIPE

MEDITERRANEAN CHICKPEA SALAD

Description of the Meal: Indulge in the vibrant flavors of the Mediterranean with this refreshing Chickpea Salad. This light and nutritious salad combines the freshness of vegetables with the hearty goodness of chickpeas, providing a satisfying meal that's perfect for any occasion.

Ingredients:

- 2 cups canned chickpeas, drained and rinsed
- 1 cucumber, diced
- 1 cup cherry tomatoes, halved
- 1 red onion, finely chopped
- 1/2 cup feta cheese, crumbled
- 1/4 cup fresh parsley, chopped
- 3 tablespoons extra-virgin olive oil
- 2 tablespoons lemon juice
- 2 cloves garlic, minced
- Salt and pepper to taste

Instructions:

1. In a large bowl, combine the chickpeas, cucumber,

cherry tomatoes, red onion, and feta cheese.

2. In a separate small bowl, whisk together the olive oil, lemon juice, and minced garlic. Season with salt and pepper to taste.

3. Pour the dressing over the salad and toss to coat the ingredients evenly.

4. Sprinkle the fresh parsley over the top for a burst of color and flavor.

5. Serve chilled and enjoy your Mediterranean Chickpea Salad!

Nutritional Information:

- Calories: 320

- Protein: 12g

- Carbohydrates: 35g

- Fat: 15g

- Fiber: 8g

QUINOA AND VEGETABLE STIR-FRY

Description of the Meal: Quinoa and Vegetable Stir-Fry is a delightful combination of fluffy quinoa and an array of colorful vegetables, stir-fried to perfection. This healthy dish is not only visually appealing but also a burst of flavors and textures.

Ingredients:

- 1 cup quinoa

- 2 cups water

- 2 tablespoons soy sauce

- 1 tablespoon sesame oil

- 1 cup broccoli florets
- 1 cup bell peppers, thinly sliced
- 1 cup snap peas
- 1 carrot, julienned
- 1 cup tofu, cubed
- 2 cloves garlic, minced
- 1 teaspoon ginger, grated
- Sesame seeds for garnish
- Green onions, chopped, for garnish

Instructions:

1. Rinse the quinoa under cold water. In a medium saucepan, combine quinoa and water. Bring to a boil, then reduce heat, cover, and simmer for about 15 minutes or until all the water is absorbed. Fluff with a fork.

2. In a small bowl, mix soy sauce and sesame oil. Set aside.

3. Heat a wok or large skillet over medium-high heat. Add a little oil and stir-fry the garlic and ginger until fragrant.

4. Add tofu and stir-fry until golden. Remove from the wok and set aside.

5. In the same wok, add more oil if needed, and stir-fry the vegetables until they are tender-crisp.

6. Return the tofu to the wok, add cooked quinoa, and pour the soy sauce mixture over the top. Stir-fry for a few more minutes.

7. Serve hot, garnished with sesame seeds and chopped green onions.

Nutritional Information:

- Calories: 380
- Protein: 14g
- Carbohydrates: 55g
- Fat: 10g
- Fiber: 7g

LENTIL SOUP

Description of the Meal: Lentil Soup is a warm and comforting dish that's both hearty and healthy. This flavorful soup is packed with protein and is perfect for a chilly day or whenever you're in need of some nourishing comfort.

Ingredients:

- 1 cup green or brown lentils, rinsed
- 1 onion, chopped
- 2 carrots, chopped
- 2 celery stalks, chopped
- 3 cloves garlic, minced
- 1 can diced tomatoes
- 6 cups vegetable broth
- 1 teaspoon cumin
- 1/2 teaspoon paprika
- Salt and pepper to taste
- Fresh parsley for garnish

Instructions:

1. In a large pot, sauté the chopped onion, carrots, and celery until they start to soften.

2. Add the minced garlic and sauté for another minute.

3. Stir in the lentils, diced tomatoes, vegetable broth, cumin, and paprika. Season with salt and pepper.

4. Bring the soup to a boil, then reduce the heat to a simmer. Cover and cook for about 25-30 minutes, or until the lentils are tender.

5. Garnish with fresh parsley before serving.

Nutritional Information:

- Calories: 250
- Protein: 15g
- Carbohydrates: 40g
- Fat: 2g
- Fiber: 8g

GRILLED SALMON WITH DILL SAUCE

Description of the Meal: Grilled Salmon with Dill Sauce is an elegant and flavorful dish that's perfect for special occasions or when you want to treat yourself. The succulent salmon, perfectly grilled, and the creamy dill sauce create a harmonious combination of taste and texture.

Ingredients:

- 4 salmon fillets
- 2 tablespoons olive oil

- Salt and pepper to taste
- 1/4 cup Greek yogurt
- 2 tablespoons mayonnaise
- 1 tablespoon fresh dill, chopped
- 1 clove garlic, minced
- 1 tablespoon lemon juice

Instructions:

1. Preheat the grill to medium-high heat.
2. Brush the salmon fillets with olive oil and season with salt and pepper.
3. Grill the salmon for about 4-5 minutes on each side, or until it flakes easily with a fork.
4. While the salmon is grilling, prepare the dill sauce. In a small bowl, combine Greek yogurt, mayonnaise, fresh dill, minced garlic, and lemon juice. Mix well.
5. Serve the grilled salmon with a dollop of dill sauce on top.

Nutritional Information:

- Calories: 320
- Protein: 28g
- Carbohydrates: 2g
- Fat: 21g
- Fiber: 0g

RATATOUILLE

Description of the Meal: Ratatouille is a classic French dish that's a celebration of vibrant, seasonal vegetables. This flavorful stew combines eggplant, zucchini, bell peppers, and tomatoes, resulting in a wholesome and colorful dish that's as pleasing to the eyes as it is to the palate.

Ingredients:

- 1 eggplant, diced
- 2 zucchinis, sliced
- 2 bell peppers, diced
- 4 tomatoes, chopped
- 1 onion, sliced
- 3 cloves garlic, minced
- 2 tablespoons olive oil
- 1 teaspoon dried thyme
- 1 teaspoon dried basil
- Salt and pepper to taste
- Fresh basil for garnish

Instructions:

1. In a large skillet, heat the olive oil over medium heat. Add the onion and garlic and sauté until fragrant.

2. Add the diced eggplant, zucchinis, and bell peppers. Cook until they start to soften.

3. Stir in the chopped tomatoes, dried thyme, and dried basil. Season with salt and pepper.

4. Reduce the heat, cover the skillet, and let it simmer for about 20-25 minutes, or until the vegetables are tender.

5. Garnish with fresh basil before serving.

Nutritional Information:

- Calories: 180

- Protein: 4g

- Carbohydrates: 28g

- Fat: 7g

- Fiber: 9g

STUFFED BELL PEPPERS

Description of the Meal: Stuffed Bell Peppers are a delightful fusion of flavors and textures. These vibrant peppers serve as nature's edible bowls, filled with a savory, fragrant mixture that's sure to tantalize your taste buds.

Ingredients:

- 4 large bell peppers (any color)

- 1 pound ground turkey

- 1 cup cooked quinoa

- 1 small onion, finely chopped

- 2 cloves garlic, minced

- 1 can diced tomatoes

- 1 cup shredded mozzarella cheese

- 1 teaspoon cumin

- Salt and pepper to taste

Instructions:

1. Preheat your oven to 375°F (190°C).

2. Cut the tops off the bell peppers and remove the

seeds and membranes.

3. In a large skillet, brown the ground turkey over medium heat, breaking it into small pieces. Add the onion and garlic, and sauté until fragrant.

4. Stir in the cooked quinoa, diced tomatoes, cumin, salt, and pepper. Cook for an additional 5 minutes.

5. Carefully stuff each bell pepper with the turkey and quinoa mixture.

6. Place the stuffed peppers in a baking dish and top each with a generous amount of mozzarella cheese.

7. Cover the dish with aluminum foil and bake for 25-30 minutes, or until the peppers are tender.

8. Remove the foil and bake for an additional 5-10 minutes until the cheese is golden and bubbly.

9. Serve hot and enjoy!

Nutritional Information:

- Calories: 320 per serving
- Protein: 26g
- Carbohydrates: 26g
- Fat: 12g
- Fiber: 5g

GREEK SALAD

Description of the Meal: Greek Salad is a refreshing, vibrant dish that captures the essence of Mediterranean cuisine. It's a colorful medley of fresh vegetables, olives, and feta cheese, all drizzled with a zesty dressing.

Ingredients:

- 2 large cucumbers, diced
- 4 ripe tomatoes, chopped
- 1 red onion, thinly sliced
- 1 cup Kalamata olives, pitted
- 1 cup crumbled feta cheese
- 1/4 cup extra-virgin olive oil
- 2 tablespoons red wine vinegar
- 1 teaspoon dried oregano
- Salt and pepper to taste

Instructions:

1. In a large bowl, combine cucumbers, tomatoes, red onion, olives, and feta cheese.
2. In a separate bowl, whisk together olive oil, red wine vinegar, dried oregano, salt, and pepper.
3. Drizzle the dressing over the salad and toss to combine.
4. Refrigerate for 30 minutes to allow the flavors to meld.
5. Serve as a refreshing side dish or add grilled chicken or shrimp for a complete meal.

Nutritional Information:

- Calories: 250 per serving
- Protein: 7g
- Carbohydrates: 12g
- Fat: 20g
- Fiber: 4g

TOFU AND VEGETABLE KEBABS

Description of the Meal: Tofu and Vegetable Kebabs are a vegan delight that's perfect for grilling season. These skewers feature marinated tofu and a colorful array of fresh vegetables, making them a healthy and satisfying choice.

Ingredients:

- 1 block extra-firm tofu, cubed
- 1 red bell pepper, cut into chunks
- 1 green bell pepper, cut into chunks
- 1 zucchini, sliced
- 1 red onion, cut into wedges
- 8 cherry tomatoes
- 1/4 cup olive oil
- 2 tablespoons soy sauce
- 2 cloves garlic, minced
- 1 teaspoon paprika
- Salt and pepper to taste

Instructions:

1. In a bowl, whisk together olive oil, soy sauce, garlic, paprika, salt, and pepper to create the marinade.

2. Thread the tofu and vegetables onto skewers, alternating colors for a visually appealing presentation.

3. Brush the kebabs with the marinade and let them sit for 15 minutes to soak up the flavors.

4. Preheat your grill to medium-high heat.

5. Grill the kebabs for about 10-12 minutes, turning occasionally, until they are nicely charred and the tofu is heated through.

6. Serve with your favorite dipping sauce or over a bed of cooked quinoa.

Nutritional Information:

- Calories: 280 per serving
- Protein: 15g
- Carbohydrates: 12g
- Fat: 20g
- Fiber: 4g

HUMMUS AND VEGGIE PLATTER

Description of the Meal: Hummus and Veggie Platter is a satisfying and wholesome snack or appetizer. Creamy hummus pairs perfectly with a colorful array of fresh, crunchy vegetables for a delightful combination of flavors and textures.

Ingredients:

- 1 cup store-bought or homemade hummus
- 1 cucumber, sliced
- 2 carrots, cut into sticks
- 1 red bell pepper, sliced
- 1 cup cherry tomatoes
- 1 cup broccoli florets
- 1 cup cauliflower florets

- 1/4 cup pitted black olives

- 1/4 cup baby spinach leaves

Instructions:

1. Arrange the hummus in the center of a large serving platter.

2. Surround the hummus with the sliced cucumber, carrot sticks, red bell pepper slices, cherry tomatoes, broccoli florets, cauliflower florets, and black olives.

3. Garnish with a handful of baby spinach leaves for an extra burst of color.

4. Serve with pita bread, crackers, or breadsticks for dipping.

Nutritional Information:

- Calories: 180 per serving

- Protein: 6g

- Carbohydrates: 20g

- Fat: 8g

- Fiber: 6g

BLACK BEAN AND CORN SALAD

Description of the Meal: Black Bean and Corn Salad is a zesty and flavorful dish that's both nutritious and delicious. This salad combines the earthiness of black beans with the sweetness of corn, creating a satisfying and colorful meal.

Ingredients:

- 1 can black beans, drained and rinsed

- 2 cups corn kernels (fresh, frozen, or canned)
- 1 red bell pepper, diced
- 1/2 red onion, finely chopped
- 1/4 cup fresh cilantro, chopped
- 2 tablespoons lime juice
- 2 tablespoons olive oil
- 1 teaspoon chili powder
- Salt and pepper to taste

Instructions:

1. In a large bowl, combine black beans, corn, red bell pepper, red onion, and fresh cilantro.
2. In a separate small bowl, whisk together lime juice, olive oil, chili powder, salt, and pepper.
3. Pour the dressing over the salad and toss to combine.
4. Refrigerate for at least 30 minutes before serving to allow the flavors to meld.
5. Serve as a side dish, on top of grilled chicken, or as a filling for tacos.

Nutritional Information:

- Calories: 180 per serving
- Protein: 6g
- Carbohydrates: 29g
- Fat: 5g
- Fiber: 7g

SWEET POTATO AND CHICKPEA CURRY

Description of the Meal: This hearty Sweet Potato and Chickpea Curry is a delightful fusion of flavors and textures. It combines the sweetness of sweet potatoes with the nuttiness of chickpeas, all enveloped in a fragrant, spiced curry sauce.

Ingredients:

- 2 large sweet potatoes, peeled and diced
- 1 can of chickpeas, drained and rinsed
- 1 onion, finely chopped
- 3 cloves of garlic, minced
- 1 can of diced tomatoes
- 2 tablespoons of curry powder
- 1 teaspoon of cumin
- 1 teaspoon of turmeric
- 1/2 teaspoon of red pepper flakes (adjust to taste)
- 1 can of coconut milk
- Salt and pepper to taste
- Fresh cilantro for garnish
- Cooked rice for serving

Instructions:

1. Heat some oil in a large pan over medium heat. Add the chopped onion and garlic. Sauté until they become translucent.

2. Add the curry powder, cumin, turmeric, and red pepper flakes. Stir for a minute to release the spices' flavors.

3. Add the sweet potato cubes and chickpeas. Mix them well with the spices.

4. Pour in the diced tomatoes and coconut milk. Season with salt and pepper.

5. Cover the pan and simmer for 20-25 minutes or until the sweet potatoes are tender.

6. Serve the Sweet Potato and Chickpea Curry over cooked rice, garnished with fresh cilantro.

Nutritional Information:

- Calories: 350

- Carbohydrates: 55g

- Protein: 10g

- Fat: 10g

- Fiber: 9g

GREEK LENTIL SALAD

Description of the Meal: The Greek Lentil Salad is a refreshing and nutritious dish that's perfect for a light meal. It's a delightful blend of lentils, fresh vegetables, and tangy feta cheese, all drizzled with a zesty Greek dressing.

Ingredients:

- 1 cup of green or brown lentils, cooked and cooled

- 1 cucumber, diced

- 1 cup of cherry tomatoes, halved

- 1 red onion, finely sliced

- 1/2 cup of crumbled feta cheese

- 1/4 cup of Kalamata olives, pitted

- Fresh parsley, chopped for garnish

Instructions:

1. In a large bowl, combine the cooked and cooled lentils, diced cucumber, halved cherry tomatoes, and sliced red onion.

2. Add the crumbled feta cheese and Kalamata olives to the salad.

3. Drizzle the zesty Greek dressing over the salad and toss to combine.

4. Garnish with fresh chopped parsley.

Nutritional Information:

- Calories: 300

- Carbohydrates: 45g

- Protein: 15g

- Fat: 8g

- Fiber: 10g

SPINACH AND MUSHROOM QUICHE

Description of the Meal: The Spinach and Mushroom Quiche is a savory delight. It's a flaky pastry crust filled with a creamy mixture of eggs, spinach, sautéed mushrooms, and gooey cheese.

Ingredients:

- 1 prepared pie crust

- 1 cup of fresh spinach, chopped
- 1 cup of mushrooms, sliced
- 1 cup of shredded Swiss cheese
- 4 large eggs
- 1 cup of milk
- 1/2 teaspoon of salt
- 1/4 teaspoon of black pepper
- 1/4 teaspoon of nutmeg

Instructions:

1. Preheat your oven to 375°F (190°C).
2. In a skillet, sauté the sliced mushrooms until they're tender. Add the chopped spinach and sauté until wilted. Set aside to cool.
3. In a bowl, whisk together the eggs, milk, salt, pepper, and nutmeg.
4. Place the pie crust in a pie dish and sprinkle half of the shredded Swiss cheese on the bottom.
5. Add the sautéed mushroom and spinach mixture.
6. Pour the egg mixture over the vegetables.
7. Sprinkle the remaining cheese on top.
8. Bake in the preheated oven for 35-40 minutes or until the quiche is set and golden brown.
9. Let it cool for a few minutes before slicing and serving.

Nutritional Information:

- Calories: 280

- Carbohydrates: 18g

- Protein: 14g

- Fat: 18g

- Fiber: 2g

BROWN RICE BOWL WITH STEAMED GREENS

Description of the Meal: The Brown Rice Bowl with Steamed Greens is a wholesome and nutritious bowl that combines the goodness of brown rice with a variety of steamed greens. It's a simple yet satisfying dish.

Ingredients:

- 2 cups of cooked brown rice

- 2 cups of mixed steamed greens (e.g., broccoli, kale, and green beans)

- 1/4 cup of toasted almonds

- 2 tablespoons of soy sauce

- 1 tablespoon of sesame oil

- Sesame seeds for garnish

Instructions:

1. Prepare the brown rice according to package instructions and set aside.

2. Steam a mix of greens until they're tender but still vibrant.

3. In a bowl, combine the steamed greens with the cooked brown rice.

4. Drizzle soy sauce and sesame oil over the rice and greens, and toss to combine.

5. Top the bowl with toasted almonds and a sprinkle of sesame seeds.

Nutritional Information:

- Calories: 400

- Carbohydrates: 70g

- Protein: 12g

- Fat: 10g

- Fiber: 8g

VEGETABLE TAGINE

Description of the Meal: The Vegetable Tagine is a Moroccan-inspired stew that's bursting with flavors. It's a medley of vegetables, dried fruits, and warm spices, slow-cooked to perfection.

Ingredients:

- 2 tablespoons of olive oil

- 1 onion, chopped

- 2 cloves of garlic, minced

- 2 carrots, sliced

- 2 zucchinis, diced

- 1 bell pepper, chopped

- 1 can of chickpeas, drained

- 1/2 cup of dried apricots, chopped

- 1/2 cup of raisins

- 2 teaspoons of ground cumin

- 1 teaspoon of ground cinnamon
- 1 teaspoon of paprika
- 1/2 teaspoon of ground coriander
- 1/4 teaspoon of cayenne pepper (adjust to taste)
- 1 can of diced tomatoes
- 2 cups of vegetable broth
- Salt and pepper to taste
- Fresh cilantro for garnish

Instructions:

1. In a large, deep pan, heat olive oil over medium heat. Add chopped onion and minced garlic. Sauté until fragrant.

2. Add carrots, zucchinis, and bell pepper. Stir and cook for a few minutes.

3. Add chickpeas, dried apricots, and raisins. Mix well.

4. Sprinkle the ground cumin, cinnamon, paprika, coriander, and cayenne pepper. Stir to coat the vegetables and chickpeas in the spices.

5. Pour in the diced tomatoes and vegetable broth. Season with salt and pepper.

6. Cover the pan and simmer for 30-40 minutes until the vegetables are tender and the sauce has thickened.

7. Serve the Vegetable Tagine over couscous or rice, garnished with fresh cilantro.

Nutritional Information:

- Calories: 320
- Carbohydrates: 60g
- Protein: 10g
- Fat: 7g
- Fiber: 9g

CHAPTER NINE

CONCLUSION

RECAP OF THE KEY TAKEAWAYS FROM THE BLUE ZONE DIET COOKBOOK.

The Blue Zone diet, inspired by regions where people live longer, healthier lives, offers a treasure trove of wisdom for anyone seeking to improve their well-being through nutrition. In this recap, we'll delve into some key takeaways from the Blue Zone diet cookbook.

1. Plant-Based Dominance

One of the fundamental principles of the Blue Zone diet is the predominance of plant-based foods. These regions emphasize the consumption of vegetables, fruits, legumes, and whole grains. Plant-based diets are rich in vitamins, minerals, and antioxidants, which promote overall health and longevity.

2. Lean Protein Sources

While the Blue Zone diet primarily consists of plant-based foods, it also includes lean protein sources like fish and poultry in moderation. These provide essential amino acids and omega-3 fatty acids, supporting muscle health and reducing the risk of chronic diseases.

3. Minimal Processed Foods

Processed foods are limited in the Blue Zone diet. These regions prioritize natural, unprocessed ingredients. This approach helps reduce the intake of unhealthy additives, excessive salt, and refined sugars, which are associated with various health issues.

4. Mindful Eating

The Blue Zone communities practice mindful eating, savoring each bite and paying attention to hunger and fullness cues. This practice encourages a healthier relationship with food, preventing overeating and promoting better digestion.

5. Social Connection

Sharing meals with loved ones is a cornerstone of the Blue Zone lifestyle. Strong social connections and communal dining contribute to reduced stress levels and increased happiness, both of which are linked to longevity.

6. Moderate Wine Consumption

In some Blue Zones, moderate wine consumption is a common practice, especially red wine. It's believed to provide heart-healthy benefits due to its antioxidants, such as resveratrol. However, it's crucial to consume alcohol in moderation to reap the potential benefits without the risks.

7. Fasting Traditions

Intermittent fasting is another intriguing aspect of the Blue Zone diet. Some communities incorporate periods of fasting or caloric restriction into their routines, which may promote metabolic health and longevity.

8. Hydration with Water

Staying hydrated with water is essential in Blue Zone regions. They prioritize water over sugary beverages, which helps maintain overall health and well-being.

9. A Sense of Purpose

Beyond diet, Blue Zone residents often share a strong sense of purpose and belonging. Having a reason to get up in the morning and staying socially engaged contribute to their overall vitality.

Encouragement to embark on a healthier lifestyle journey.

Embarking on a healthier lifestyle journey is a decision that can lead to a more fulfilling and longer life. Here's some encouragement to help you take those first steps towards a healthier you.

1. Set Realistic Goals

Begin with achievable, small goals. Whether it's adding an extra serving of vegetables to your meals or going for a short walk each day, setting realistic targets ensures you won't feel overwhelmed.

2. Find Your Motivation

Identify the reasons why you want to lead a healthier lifestyle. Whether it's to have more energy, reduce the risk of chronic diseases, or simply feel better in your own skin, knowing your motivation can help you stay committed.

3. Embrace Variety

Don't limit yourself to a rigid diet. Explore different foods, recipes, and exercise routines to keep things interesting. Variety not only makes your journey enjoyable but also ensures you get a wide range of nutrients.

4. Seek Support

Enlist the support of friends, family, or a support group.

Sharing your goals and progress with others can provide motivation and accountability.

5. Practice Mindfulness

Mindfulness can help you become more aware of your habits and make healthier choices. Pay attention to what you eat and how it makes you feel, both physically and emotionally.

6. Be Patient

Healthy lifestyle changes take time. Don't be discouraged by setbacks or slow progress. Celebrate your small victories along the way, as they add up to significant improvements over time.

7. Stay Informed

Educate yourself about nutrition, exercise, and wellness. Knowledge empowers you to make informed choices and adapt your lifestyle to suit your individual needs.

8. Prioritize Sleep

A good night's sleep is essential for overall health. Ensure you get enough quality sleep to support your body's repair and regeneration processes.

9. Stay Consistent

Consistency is key to long-term success. Make healthy choices a habit by integrating them into your daily routine.

Final thoughts on the long-term advantages of the Blue Zone diet.

In conclusion, adopting the principles of the Blue Zone diet can lead to numerous long-term advantages for your health and well-being.

1. Increased Lifespan

The Blue Zone diet, with its focus on plant-based foods and minimal processed items, has been associated with longer lifespans. It reduces the risk of chronic diseases and supports overall vitality.

2. Enhanced Heart Health

The inclusion of lean proteins and moderate wine consumption, particularly red wine, can promote heart health by reducing the risk of heart disease and improving cardiovascular function.

3. Weight Management

The emphasis on natural, nutrient-dense foods and mindful eating can aid in weight management and reduce the risk of obesity, a significant contributor to various health issues.

4. Better Mental Health

The social connections, sense of purpose, and mindfulness practices within Blue Zone communities contribute to improved mental well-being and lower stress levels.

5. Balanced Nutrition

The Blue Zone diet provides a balanced and diverse range of nutrients, ensuring that you receive essential vitamins and minerals for optimal health.

6. Enhanced Quality of Life

By following the Blue Zone diet and lifestyle, you can experience an enhanced quality of life, characterized by better physical health, emotional well-being, and longevity.

Incorporating the key takeaways from the Blue Zone diet

into your life and embarking on a journey towards a healthier lifestyle can lead to a happier, more fulfilling, and longer life. So, take that first step today and savor the benefits of a well-nourished, vibrant existence.